Why health care costs so much: The Solution – Consumers

By Greg Dattilo, CEBS
Dave Racer, MLitt

Alethos Press LLC
St. Paul, MN

ALETHOS PRESS LLC
PO Box 600160
St. Paul, MN 55106

Why Health Care Costs So Much: The Solution - Consumers

ISBN 978-0-9777534-3-7

Artwork by Tom Foty:
http://tomfotyart.com

Printed in the U.S.A. by
Bethany Press International,
Bloomington, MN

http://www.alethospress.com/whycost.htm
http://www.freemarkethealthcare.com

10 9 8 7 6 5 4 3 2 1

TABLE OF CONTENTS

INTRODUCTION

HEALING U.S. HEALTH CARE

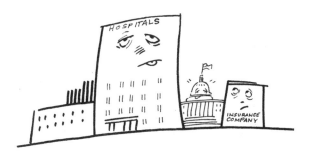

You are hearing that the United States health care system is in a crisis, if not terminally ill. This book shows you how to heal it.

This book is about understanding *why* health care costs so much, and how *you* have the power to change it. You change it by adopting new behaviors, about how you spend health care dollars, and how you care for your own body. The truth is that the combined behavior of each of us determines the quality and cost of health care, for good or for bad.

In our first book, *Your Health Matters: What you need to know about U.S. health care,*[1] we wrote how the U.S. health system is unique in the world. We showed that the U.S. has the world's most advanced and expensive health care. The U.S. is unique in that we provide access

---

[1] Dattilo, G.; Racer, D. (2006) *Your Health Matters: What you need to know about US health care*. Alethos Press LLC, St. Paul, MN,

to care for every conceivable type of health problem for all U.S. residents.

One section of *Your Health Matters* describes the health systems of five modern, foreign nations. We show how their national governments dictate how individuals receive health care. While they want you to believe everyone has access to affordable health care, that is not necessarily true. They often ration care for people with life-threatening conditions, and are beset by long wait times for vital health services. Yet, their residents pay enormous taxes to support this "free" care.

Many foreign governments have begun allowing residents to opt out of the government health system for private, voluntary health insurance. Canadians spitefully call this "Americanizing Canadian health care."

We don't want to Americanize *Canadian* health care, we want to Americanize *American* health care. This means putting you in charge of your own life and money. It means creating a system where doctors, hospitals, and insurance companies must compete for your health care dollars.

We believe that given the right tools and information, *you* will heal the system.

BUT HOW CAN *YOU* HEAL THE HEALTH CARE SYSTEM?

There are two ways that you can reduce the cost of health care – be healthier and spend less.

Healthier people need less health care. This is true for today, and over a lifetime. There is universal agreement that each of us need to become healthier to help reduce health spending. This is called wellness. Many *other* books and websites are devoted to wellness, and we urge you to take the time to learn about it. It is a key element in solving the high cost of health care.

The larger problem is that few people understand the reasons we pay so much for health care.

We believe that if you make more informed choices about paying for health care, you will also make healthier lifestyle choices. Which comes first? Wellness and then reduced spending? Or more careful spending and then wellness? Does it really matter? They are both necessary.

This book explains why health care costs so much, and then it shows how you are the solution. You might say this book will make you healthier and wealthier.

CHAPTER I

THIS IS ONE EXAMPLE OF WHY HEALTH CARE COSTS SO MUCH

Medicare is the U.S. government health plan that primarily covers people 65 and older.

In 2006, Medicare reported that U.S. hospitals billed Medicare on average, 308 percent more than the actual Medicare payments to those hospitals (for the 31 most common procedures). To illustrate, for one type of heart operation, Medicare reimbursed the hospitals an average of $39,361; *but the hospitals billed Medicare $124,561 for the same operation![2]* (To view this government document go to: http://www.freemarkethealthcare.com/why-cost.htm)

Why would hospitals bill Medicare three times more than what Medicare reimburses them? Doesn't this seem

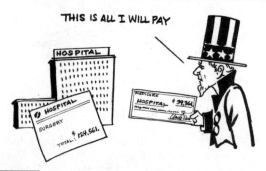

---

[2] Top 31 Hospital Procedures by DRG. Centers for Medicare and Medicaid Services. 2008. Data is drawn from 2005. Retrieved from http://www.cms.gov on July 25, 2008.

outrageous? Yet, this is the "gotcha" game that hospitals have played for years, and a key reason why health care costs so much.

The amount hospitals bill Medicare is usually the same that hospitals bill insurance companies and private individuals. Is this why uninsured people often can't afford their hospital bills? And why should *anyone* be forced to pay $124,561 for surgery – the gotcha price – that people on Medicare can get for $39,361?

In these pages, we will show that people like you, armed with common sense and the willingness to ask the "consumerized question," will have the ability to change this "gotcha" system.

Here is what we mean by the "gotcha" system; it is when you use health care services and pay far more than you need to pay, but you do not know until it's too late. The system..."gotcha."

Here is what we mean by the "consumerized" system; it is when you participate in making decisions about your own health care, and you know the cost before you decide what to do about it. Using the consumerized system vaccinates you against "gotcha."

THE HOSPITAL CHARGED
THE AUTHOR A GOTCHA PRICE

One of the authors suffered from chest pains during the summer of 2008. As a result, his doctor sent him to the hospital to take a "nuclear" heart stress test. The entire test took no more than 45 minutes.

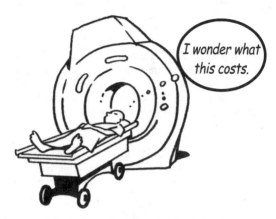

The stress test results showed he had a healthy, strong heart. The author's heart, however, nearly jumped out of his chest when he saw the bill for the stress test.

The hospital had billed the author's insurance company $6,106 for the test. The insurance company had agreed to pay the hospital only $1,188. Presumably, the hospital knows it can make a profit charging $1,188; then why did it charge $6,106? That would add $4,918 more in profit to what they accepted as payment – a whopping 414 percent more than they needed!

Normal profit for any other large purchase (cars, TVs, washing machines, etc.) is usually three to five percent, not 414 percent.

What should frighten you is this: If the author had been uninsured, the hospital would have chased him down for $6,106. That is *nearly $5,000 more than it needed to be paid*. This is the gotcha price.

The author still had lessons to learn; lessons shared in this book.

CHAPTER 2

HOW *DO* AMERICANS PAY FOR HEALTH CARE?

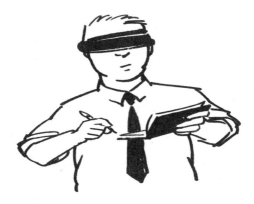

There are four primary ways Americans pay for health care:

◆ Government health care for those aged 65 and older (Medicare).

◆ Government health care for low-income people younger than 65 (Medicaid and other programs).

◆ People with private health insurance (from employers or individual insurance).

◆ People without insurance – uninsured.

Which of those four groups of people would know the cost of health care?

For those with a government-paid health plan, there is no reason to know or ask the actual cost of health care. They are insulated from the cost.

Medicare patients don't pay their own health care bills;[3] except, perhaps, for a low co-pay. Medicare and supplemental insurance pays their bills.

People who receive health care through Medicaid or other government-paid health plans do not pay their own health care bills, except for a very low co-pay. *Taxpayers pay nearly 100 percent of their bills.*

If your health insurance is provided by an employer or you buy an individual policy, wanting to know the price of health care services depends on what kind of insurance you own.

If you have a traditional health plan (HMO/PPO), you only know about co-pays. You do not know the actual cost of care. The actual cost is paid by your insurance company.

If you own a health insurance policy that primarily protects you from large, catastrophic expenses and not minor health expenses, you *will* want to know the cost of care before you receive it. You pay a good deal of the actual cost before the insurance company begins to pay.

Oddly enough, only if you are *uninsured* do you find out how much health care providers actually charge. This is because *you* have to pay the entire bill, not someone else. The sad thing is that you usually don't find out the price until after you receive the care, when it's too late to shop for a better value. *Gotcha.*

---

[3] Medicare patients pay a deductible if they have a hospital stay. If they have an extended hospital stay, they will be charged daily rates. But if they have supplemental insurance, they usually pay nothing.

NOT KNOWING THE PRICE

You may never have heart surgery, but you probably go to a doctor's office. If you have traditional prepaid health insurance with an office co-pay of $15, $20, or $25, that is all you pay. You have no reason to ask the total price of the office visit because your prepaid insurance will pay the rest. But you really *do* have a reason to ask; the more the doctor charges your insurance company, the more you will have to pay in future higher premiums.

You would be more motivated to know the price if your insurance only paid the *first* $15, $20, or $25 for an office visit and *you* paid the rest. You would want to know the *actual* price the doctor charges.

KNOWING THE PRICE - A HUGE SAVINGS

Many people take cholesterol-reducing drugs. One of the most popular is simvastatin. Many drug companies manufacture it today. Merck created simvastatin in 1991, and sells it under the *brand name* Zocor.

Zocor sells for as much as $1,786 a year for the 20 mg dose.[4] If you have a prescription co-pay of $20 per month, the cost makes little difference to you because

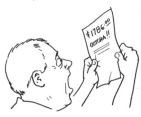

your cost would be limited to $240 a year. The insurance company pays the difference: $1,546. To pay *their* share, the insurance company increases your premium along with everyone else's. Gotcha.

But if *you* had to pay the *full* price, you might opt for simvastatin made by a different manufacturer that pro-

---

[4] Quoted by phone by a pharmacist at a national pharmaceutical chain on August 8, 2008.

[5] Quoted from Internet tables for a national discount chain store, August 8, 2008.

duces the same drug: This is called a generic. Generic manufacturers keep their prices as low as possible.

Instead of buying Zocor, you could buy generic simvastatin. For 20 mg, this could cut your cost to $38 a year[5] – a whopping savings of 97.9 percent! If you buy generic

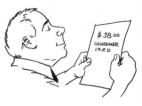

simvastatin, your insurance company saves $1,546, and you save $202. As a result, your insurance premium would be stable. This is called consumerism. (Later on we will show you how to reduce the price by *another 35 percent*.)

This is an example of why health care costs so much; when it's someone else's money, people spend more, and this creates waste. How would you change your health purchasing behavior if you paid the full price, or half the price, or even if you *knew* the price?

How could anyone pay only *half* the price for health care?

In 1960, Americans paid 48 percent of their doctor and hospital bill directly to the provider (doctor or hospital). The insurance company, or in a small number of cases a government program, paid the rest of the bill. Uninsured people paid for their own health care, or received it from charitable clinics and county hospitals.

By 2006, individuals paid only *12 percent* of their health care bills from their own pocket. Someone else, government or insurance, paid the other 88 percent.

What was the buying behavior when Americans paid their own bills?

The 1960 health care shopper behaved like a consumer. Many had a family doctor to whom they were loyal. They called the doctor when they felt it was necessary. They received quality health care, and as much as they believed they needed. They had a financial incentive to be careful, and to take better care of themselves. They knew the cost of their health care because they paid 48 percent of it out of their own pocket.

Rather than pay very expensive health insurance premiums as we do today, *they* bought affordable, major medical health insurance policies. These policies protected their assets from large financial losses as a result of a serious illness or injury, and gave them the security to know that their health needs would be met.

Those 1960 doctors had to charge a reasonable price that people felt gave them value for services received. Doctors focused on pleasing the patient, because the patient paid them, unlike today. Today, the doctor has to please the government or the insurance company, because they get paid by them.

If those 1960s Americans could purchase health care on their own, how much better equipped are people today? Whether aided by an insurance agent, website, care coordinator, doctor, some other specialist, or just on your own, you are *more* than capable of navigating the purchase of health care. And when *you* are in charge you can save yourself a lot of money *and* be healthier.

But, we lack the most important information that drives consumer behavior; the price of health care services. How did we go from knowing the price, to not knowing the price?

CHAPTER 3:

GOOD MOTIVES WITH UNINTENDED CONSEQUENCES

From the days when we bought health insurance to protect ourselves from the cost of major medical expenses, we have come to the place where we expect our health insurance to pay for everything. From affordable health insurance, we now have very expensive prepaid health care. This has changed our health purchasing behavior. How did this happen? This story will help explain it.

Let's say that seven years ago your auto insurance agent gave you great news: Your auto policy, for which
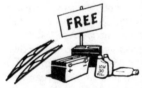
you have never had a claim, would now include *prepaid auto maintenance*. It would cover the cost of windshield wipers, oil changes and batteries. You would receive all these extra benefits, and still have coverage in case you have an accident. The best news is that these new benefits would be *free*; your insurance premium stayed the same.

"The car insurance companies are doing this to attract good drivers who are uninsured to buy auto insurance," your agent explained.

Within weeks, news reported that thousands of previously uninsured auto owners had signed up: They really liked the new prepaid maintenance coverage. Now they saw a way to get some of their insurance premium back without having an accident. Before, they never expected to collect on car insurance, but now they could get these maintenance services for "free." Since prepaid maintenance paid for routine car care, the consumer lost concern about price: Their insurance *entitled* them to these maintenance services.

YEAR TWO – GREAT BARGAIN, SIGN ME UP!

"I have some bad news and some good news," your agent said a year later. "The bad news is that your insurance premium went up, but here is the good news, and I think you're going to like it."

He said you could add prepaid tire coverage to your prepaid maintenance coverage for just $60 a year. If you needed new tires, you could buy any brand you wanted, and all you had to pay was a $10 co-pay for each tire.

"Sign me up," you said.

The next day you drove to Dr. Tom's Tires, where you've done business for 20 years. You had him change the oil and install new windshield wipers. You also had him install the most expensive tires: $110 each. With your $60 prepaid tire insurance premium and $40 in co-pays, you bought $440 worth of tires for $100 – a great deal!

The great prepaid tire insurance deal caught on with a lot of people. Then the insurance company started losing money paying their share of the bill. Far too many people wanted a bargain and began using their prepaid tire insurance. The insurance company took a $340 loss on each set of tires.

YEAR THREE – GREAT BARGAIN
FOR LESS FREEDOM TO CHOOSE

"Well once again, good news and bad news," your agent said. "You can still buy any tire you want, but the insurance company says you have to use Network Tire Shops (NTS)." The Network shops had agreed to accept a reduced payment for tires, batteries, oil changes, and wipers from the insurance companies.

You looked in the NTS Directory to see if it included Dr. Tom's Tires. It didn't. Now you had to make a decision: You could still choose to go to Dr. Tom's Tires and not be covered by your insurance, but you would have to pay the full price. Or, you could sign up at an NTS shop and just pay your $10 co-pay per tire. This meant breaking a long time relationship with Dr. Tom's, and you really didn't like it. *But I prepaid for the coverage*, you reasoned, *I should get my money back.* You chose the NTS shop.

GREAT BARGAIN FOR LESS DECISION-MAKING

You chose to go to Metro Tire Supply, an NTS shop and learned a lesson about managed prepaid maintenance car care. The tire installer had to get permission from your insurance company manager before installing the new tires. This bothered you, but since you only had to pay $10 a tire you put up with it.

Your insurance company agreed to allow you to get new tires, but not the new design. Furthermore, they would only replace the *front* tires this year. You spent a few minutes thinking about this: The cost of tires had gone up, you still only paid the co-pay, and the prepaid premium had remained affordable. You felt entitled to four tires, but even getting two was a good deal. Besides, you were still able to get regular oil changes and new wipers for free.

YEAR FOUR – NO HEALTHY COMPETI- TION; ONE-SIDED MONOPOLY

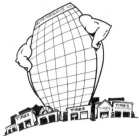

The fourth year, the prepaid tire and mainte- nance insurance was no longer a good deal for the insurance company; they were losing money. The insurance company had to make a decision – raise your premium and co-pay, or negotiate a larger discount with the Network Tire Shops. The in- surance companies found that negotiating was easy enough, since there were a lot of tire shops and only two insurance companies left in the area. Many tire shops needed to be in the network to attract business.

The Network shops, however, also made a discov- ery: 75 percent of their bills were paid by the two car in- surance companies. They felt forced to accept whatever the insurance company would pay to make sure they had enough customers to stay in business.

The two insurance companies controlled where their policyholders would buy tires. The Networks depended on getting those customers to their sales floor. The insur- ance companies used this power to negotiate deeper dis- counts with the Network shops; as great as 50 percent off their retail price.

The Network shops now realized they were not mak- ing a profit on sales to those with prepaid maintenance in- surance. To recoup their loss, they raised their retail prices so that those without insurance had to pay *twice as much* as those with insurance. They had shifted the cost to unin- sured people.

YEAR FIVE – NO COMPETITION, NO BARGAIN, PRICE SKYROCKETS, YOU PAY

In the fifth year you stopped to see Dr. Tom. You found that he no longer owned his store. Metro Tire Supply had bought him out. Dr. Tom told you that there were no independent tire shops left: They had been bought out or just quit.

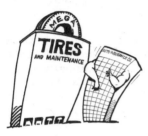

A few weeks later, you went to Metro Tire Supply and found they had also merged with other tire dealers, now called Mega Tires and Maintenance.

All the other tire shops had closed down or had been merged into Mega Tires and Maintenance. When the insurance companies were ready to negotiate a new contract with Mega, they faced a disadvantage – Mega had established a monopoly; they owned all the tire shops. Mega demanded a 75 percent increase. The two insurance companies had to pay Mega's increased price because their policyholders had nowhere else to buy tires.

Instead of telling you about the 75 percent increase that Mega demanded, the insurance company raised your premium from the $60 you *were* paying, to $150 a year, and raised your co-pay to $25 a tire. Then they added co-pays for windshield wipers, oil changes, and batteries. Unfortunately, those $110 tires had become $330 each without insurance.

You felt you had no choice but to keep paying for the prepaid tire and maintenance insurance, unwilling to take the risk to own a car without it. You knew that without insurance, the tire dealer would charge you 300 percent more than those with insurance.

YEAR SIX — WASTE ALWAYS INCREASES COST

Now that the prepaid tire and maintenance premiums had gotten more expensive, more people began to use their prepaid insurance more often, wanting to get more use out of it. They had become used to throwing away good tires, windshield wipers, and batteries, and asking for oil changes every 2,000 miles. They wanted value for their prepaid tire and maintenance premium. Policyholders felt entitled to use the prepaid coverage. Mega Tires and Maintenance, too, needed them to keep coming.

Policyholders got angry. They now paid higher premiums for less coverage. They also got tired of being turned down by the insurance company maintenance managers for the prepaid tire and maintenance coverage they believed they paid for. They said the insurance companies were heartless, and accused them of letting good cars die for no reason.

The insurance company grew frustrated with the constant bad publicity, and gave up the fight. They gave the policyholders whatever they wanted, and just raised the cost of insurance every year.

Used tires stacked up, and it meant building expensive disposal sites. Recyclers tried to keep up with the used battery supply, and sent millions of them to third world nations.

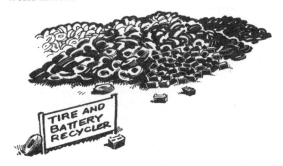

Things had gotten out of hand. A prepaid maintenance insurance crisis had developed. The cost had sky-
rocketed, tire spending had gone through the roof, and
more people began to drop insurance. The uninsured rate
became intolerable.

POLITICIANS FELT NEEDED

"Someone's got to do something," the politician said,
"and I'm the one to do it."

Some politicians pointed to
foreign governments where tires
were now being rationed. Cars
older than 15 years could no
longer get new tires. The government decided which cars
could be fixed, and which had to be scrapped. Cars that
kept breaking down lost their prepaid maintenance coverage altogether. The public became outraged.

Then, politicians added dozens of new statutes regu-
lating auto prepaid maintenance insurance. This made it
even more complicated and expensive.

"Enough! It's time to get back to letting the market
set tire prices," other politicians said. And every election
cycle, the debate raged.

CONSUMER BEHAVIOR CHANGED

In our example of auto prepaid maintenance insurance, we watched as affordable tires became unaffordable,
and fewer people could afford insurance. There were clear
reasons for all of this: Behavior changed from careful
shopping to waste and entitlement. Price gouging happened once there no longer was competition from other
tire shops as they all joined together to form a monopoly.

The moral of our story is that when someone else
pays your bill, your behavior changes. You quit being a

conscientious consumer and become captive to an *entitlement mindset*. This leads to wasteful behavior that makes insurance and services overly expensive.

America began as a nation of self-reliant individuals who understood that everything they owned had to be earned by the sweat of their brow. But modern Americans were led down the road to an entitlement mindset. Where did this entitlement mindset come from?

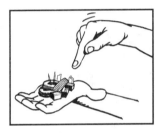

CHAPTER 4:

WORKING FOR IT OR ENTITLED TO IT?

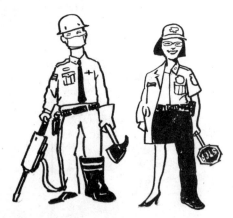

During World War II, the U.S. government placed a freeze on wages and salaries. As a response, in 1942 employers used a health insurance benefit to lure new employees, and retain current employees. The U.S. government encouraged this by making the insurance premium tax deductible to employers and tax free to employees.

Today, there are still many people who continue to work just to keep their health insurance coverage in force. This helps businesses retain experienced employees and helps reduce both the unemployed and uninsured rate.

Americans knew the value of private sector jobs. Having millions of Americans gainfully employed made us a great and strong nation. Giving employers a tax break for health insurance helped build the world's most powerful economy by encouraging work and tying health care to employment.

After 1942, if you worked for someone else in the United States there was a good chance private health insurance came with the job. Other individuals bought their own policies from their own income. If you did not work, you either paid for health care and insurance yourself, or if unable to pay for your own care, received it at a government or charitable health facility.

In contrast to the United States, other nations did not tie health insurance to employment. Instead of earning insurance at work, citizens became *entitled* to it. Every citizen had a *right* to the same health benefit, whether or not they worked. Citizens of these foreign nations bought into this idea and agreed to pay higher taxes. As a result, foreign nations tax their citizens far greater than we do in the United States. Since they paid such high taxes, people felt entitled to use their tax-paid health care systems more often. It created a behavior of entitlement and waste. *This entitlement and waste forced the government to ration health care to keep from going bankrupt.*

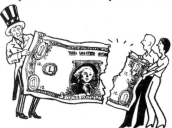

The sad thing is that wherever governments run health care, sick people find their care rationed while healthy people get all the "free" care they want. Not getting health care when you need it is an expensive way to own "free" health care.

IMPORTING HEALTH CARE FROM WESTERN EUROPE

In 1965, Congress decided that our system of private

health insurance had failed to provide the kind of broad coverage the politicians wanted for the American people. Congress imported socialized prepaid health care as an entitlement for those aged 65 and older, calling it Medicare. And Congress also created Medicaid, to pay the cost of health services for low-income people under 65.

People on Medicare and Medicaid are already enrolled in the type of socialized health systems common to Canada, France, the United Kingdom, and other industrialized nations. The greatest difference is that in the United States, there is a large private insurance system that adds nearly a trillion dollars a year to help fund health care. That means that nearly 50 percent of the total U.S. health care dollars come from private insurance. That money is in addition to what government spends from tax dollars. The result is that people on government health plans can choose from a well-stocked, nearly endless "buffet" of health services.

Those 1960s Medicare and Medicaid recipients began to feel entitled to use these new, almost free (or totally free) health services. Health care spending immediately began to spike higher by double digits.

Politicians again stepped forward. Instead of fixing Medicare and Medicaid, Congress adopted European model health plans for the *rest* of us.

Congress passed the Health Maintenance Organization (HMO) Act in 1973. As in our story about prepaid auto insurance, health care behavior changed dramatically. For the first time, people began to think that they *should* collect on health insurance. This meant going to the doctor often, using the health care services to which they now felt entitled.

Since the 1960s, politicians and activist reformers have continuously claimed that the United States is having a health care "crisis." As long as we want someone else to pay for our health care, and as long as we ask politicians to fix it, we will continue to suffer from this "crisis."

Today, most Americans do not own "health insurance." They own prepaid health care, like the prepaid tire and maintenance coverage in our example above. You may know prepaid health care as an HMO or a PPO. These types of plans encourage you to use health care services without consideration of the cost. Low co-pays actually encourage you to use more health care services because the cost seems so low.

CHAPTER 5

PREPAID HEALTH CARE

The idea behind prepaid health care was to catch diseases before they became serious and costly. Reformers believed it would reduce future health care spending: This was a great mistake. The idea ignored how it negatively changed human behavior by creating an entitlement mentality. People came to see health care as unlimited, and this resulted in overuse and waste. They quit asking how much health care cost, because their prepaid insurance covered everything under one price – the premium.

Prepaid care also rewarded poor health behavior. An insured person who chose an unhealthy lifestyle went to the doctor more often. They began feeling that the health care system could take care of any problem, and as such, they received more value for their prepaid premium.

LIKE A BUFFET DINNER

We buy prepaid health care as if it was a buffet dinner. At the buffet, we pay a single price that entitles us to eat as much as we want. This feels like a value, but it encourages wasteful and unhealthy behavior.

You measure a buffet's value by how much you pay and how many plates of food you consume. Three plates feel like three times the value of one plate. (With prepaid health care, if you go to the doctor three times instead of once, you feel as though you have received three times the value for your prepaid premium.)

"I ate four plates," your friend brags when you leave the buffet.

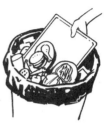

"Yes, but you threw away at least a plateful…or two," you say.

If you throw away some of the food, that seems okay; you paid for it. The fact that this creates immense waste for the restaurant is of little regard. When you come back the next time, you notice the price has gone up and you complain. Wasteful behavior drove the cost higher. (When you use a prepaid health plan more often than needed, it reinforces a behavior of waste. Wasteful behavior is common to prepaid health plans, and is passed along through higher prepaid premiums.)

"Yeah, I threw away some food, but if I ate any more I'd gain weight," your friend says. "Besides, I had to save room for the desserts."

THE HEALTH CARE BUFFET

A health care buffet includes nearly every medical and hospital service imaginable. You do not know the cost of any single service. You pay the same co-pay for a simple office visit or an extensive check-up. You "consume" it as you feel you need to, without regard to price.

With the dinner buffet, you keep going as long as the price is affordable. If it becomes too expensive, you go to a different restaurant and order *ala carte* (off the menu). When you order *ala carte* you choose among steak, chicken, or a salad because you know the *price* of each; and you order only what you want, without paying for food you do not choose to eat. You might skip the beverage, opting for a free glass of water to keep the cost down.

When you are finished with dinner, you ask for a doggy bag, making sure you have gotten the most value for your dollars.

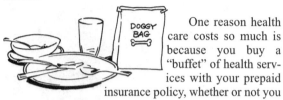

One reason health care costs so much is because you buy a "buffet" of health services with your prepaid insurance policy, whether or not you wish to. This adds as much as 40 percent (maybe more) to your health insurance premium.

What if you could order health care *ala carte*?

We think a key to healing the high cost of health care is to get rid of wasted spending, change unhealthy behaviors, and take control of your own health dollars. This is like ordering dinner *ala carte*, instead of paying for an expensive buffet filled with foods you do not need or want.

Most Americans today have prepaid health care. It requires an expensive monthly premium and covers (prepays) almost all health care expenses. As a result, the more services you use, the better the value feels to you. If you use fewer services, it feels like a poor value – and it is.

With a prepaid health plan you pay for all the extras, *plus* you pay for major medical insurance. You send a lot of money to the insurance company for this prepaid benefit – as much as 40 percent. Instead, you could save that 40 percent and buy *ala carte;* major medical insurance that will protect you from the cost of an unexpected and expensive accident or illness.

Owning a major medical health plan results in the changing of unhealthy behavior to healthy behavior. How? You save money by buying fewer health services that you do not need, and paying less for those you *do* need – *ala carte* (below, we will show you how). You also become more aware of your *physical* health, knowing that staying healthier means you will spend less for health services.

Healing U.S. health care means that we should stop paying the Gotcha Price, and begin paying the Consumerized Price. In order to do this, you start acting like a consumer. This begins with the simple question, "How much does this cost?"

HOW TO BE A HEALTH CARE CONSUMER

CHAPTER 6

How much for that stress test?

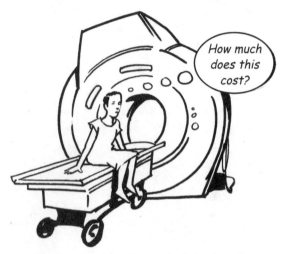

How much does this cost?

The next step is to change the behaviors that cause health care to cost so much. This starts with asking this golden question: "How much does this cost?" Yes, just ask: *"How much does this cost?"*

Why haven't people been asking how much health care costs? There is a sense that it is wrong to ask the price. It is assumed you will pay whatever the cost is for recommended treatment, regardless of the price, if you feel it will help you become healthier.

We have come to believe that it is wrong to place a dollar value on our health care. Yet, if we have no dollars left because health care becomes unaffordable, then worry and stress creates more health care problems.

We have to change our thinking about buying health care services. We need to treat *these* purchases as we would any other necessary purchase. You want to know what you are getting, why you need it, and how much it costs.

When you ask, "How much does this cost?" it naturally follows that you want to know what you are getting for the money you might have to spend. Is it worth it? Is it necessary? Are there alternatives? Asking the question creates a natural conversation with your health care provider that will lead to an informed decision about the value you will receive.

So remember: You have the right to ask the question, "How much does this cost?" and you should make a habit of it.

Don't be surprised if the doctor asks, "Why do you want to know the cost? Don't you have insurance?"

"Yes, but I don't want the premium to go higher than it is," you answer. Then ask again, "How much does this cost?"

"Well, I can't tell you because of the contract I have with your insurance company," the doctor might say.

"But it's *my* insurance. I want to know the cost of my health care." If the doctor does not tell you, you can call the insurance company to get the answer.

As a consumer, you have a right to ask the cost of your health care, and in some states the law compels the doctor or insurance company to tell you. Even if the doctor will not tell you, keep asking. The more often doctors hear the question, the more likely they will change their answer to, "Let me look it up," or, "We will get it for you."

It all starts with you repeatedly asking the question, "How much does this cost?"

IF THEY WON'T TELL YOU THE PRICE

If they won't tell you the price, they don't want you to know the price. This means that they don't want *you* to know the price!

Why would a doctor or hospital want to avoid telling you the price? Do they want to charge you the Gotcha Price? Do they want you to pay 300-500 percent more than others pay for the same services from the same doctor or hospital?

Earlier we revealed that hospitals tried to collect 308 percent more than what Medicare would pay them for the same service. Medicare refuses to pay the Gotcha Price. Medicare is not hesitant to ask "How much does this cost?" Neither should *you* be hesitant to ask.

When you make other purchases, you know the price before you pull out your checkbook or credit card. It is absurd that you are not allowed to know the price of health care before spending your money. Let us illustrate this.

Suppose that you are shopping for a house. The house you are standing in feels good to you.

"What do you think?" the realtor asks.

"I love it."

"Fine, sign this paper and it's yours." The realtor hands you a clipboard with a partially completed form under the spring clip.

"Well, how much does this house cost?" you ask.

"Why do you want to know the cost? Don't you have a mortgage company?" the realtor asks.

"Yes, I have a mortgage company," you say, "but I don't want my payment to be higher than it has to be."

"Well, I can't tell you because of the contract I have with the mortgage company," the realtor explains. "Your mortgage company says your monthly payment will be affordable. Don't worry about the purchase price."

At this point you would probably walk out the door. No one would buy a house this way. Yet health care is bought this way every day. And at times, it costs more than a house.

Now, imagine that you have moved into that house, and when you finally reviewed all the paperwork you see that you paid $200,000, and your monthly payments were barely affordable. You walk next door to an identical house to meet the neighbor who moved in the same day as you did.

"Great house," you say.

"Yup, a perfect retirement house for me," he says.

"I guess it was worth the $200,000 price," you say, trying to sound convincing.

"Oh, you paid the *Gotcha* Price," he answers.

"What do you mean the gotcha price?"

"Did your realtor tell you that they couldn't give you the price because they had a contract with the mortgage company?" he asks.

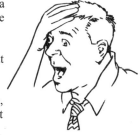

"Yes, that's exactly what happened."

"They tried that with me, too," he said. "I found out

what the house was really worth, got a different mortgage company and they wrote a check for $100,000. I paid the consumerized price, not the gotcha price!"

We agree that this house story is far-fetched. Yet, this story is not so far-fetched when it comes to how we purchase health care. Instead, this is common and even more absurd. Here is a true story from 2008:

> In Minnesota, John Roe,[6] an insured person employed by a small Minnesota company, suffered a serious illness. During a 12 month period, Roe's health care providers billed him $1,981,000 to provide health care services.

> Roe's insurance company paid the providers $597,000, covering all of Roe's health care expenses, except for a $2,500 deductible. By this, the providers showed they could make a profit accepting $597,000.

> Should we applaud the providers for giving up an additional $1,384,000 in profits to help this very sick man? Or, is it just possible that the providers made enough profit while collecting $597,000?

> If Roe had asked, "How much does this cost?" do you think the providers could have gotten away with billing him $1,981,000 when the real price was $597,000?

This is why you need to ask, "How much does this cost?" each time the doctor recommends a health service. When millions of others like you begin asking, "How much does it cost?" it will result in people like John Roe and you getting a fair and honest price for health services. It will reduce everyone's cost of health care.

So, do you want to pay the gotcha price, or the consumerized price?

---

[6] Fictitious name, but the story is true and the Explanation of Benefits is on file.

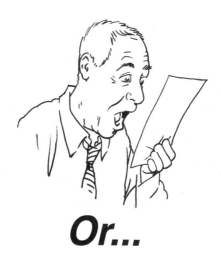

Or...

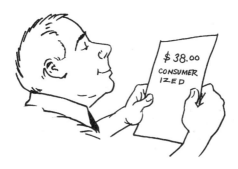

CHAPTER 7

CONSUMERIZING HEALTH CARE

If you belong to an expensive prepaid HMO, or own an expensive PPO health insurance plan, you may be less motivated to ask, "How much does this cost?" There is no instant savings from asking this question, because you have already prepaid the services and everything is inclusive. The only motivation to ask about cost is the remote possibility of some day enjoying reduced insurance premiums on these expensive health insurance plans.

What if, instead, you could keep the savings between the consumerized and gotcha price? Would you be more motivated to ask, "How much does it cost?" This kind of motivation immediately changes your behavior from wasteful to consumerized behavior.

When Dr. Jones says, "You need an MRI," you ask, "How much does it cost?"

"It depends. If you have it at the hospital it is $2,100," Dr. Jones says, "or you can go to an MRI center. It will be about $700."

"That's still a lot of money," you say. "Is there something else we can do?"

"Yes, you could try these exercises for the next month," Dr. Jones says. "That could take the strain off your back. And it costs you nothing, except time."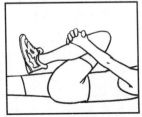

Exercising means a change of behavior, but it is one that will also reduce your cost of health care. It makes sense.

You received four immediate rewards by asking, "How much does this cost?"

1. You found out that hospitals charge three times as much as a non-hospital facility for the same service.

2. You were given choices for the treatment of your back.

3. You were given a reason to start exercising, to become healthier.

4. You saved money.

The point of this story is that when you ask "How much does this cost?" it will usually open up other, less expensive options. Asking the question is a natural way to begin a dialogue with your doctor.

COST AND VALUE ARE CLOSE COUSINS

Knowing the price of care is the starting place, but there is more you should know. The most expensive care does not mean best, and the cheapest care does not mean worst. What you pay must be related to the quality of care received – you want value for your health dollar. But value cannot be judged unless you know the price.

Lisa and Kate[7] lived in the same metropolitan area. They did not know each other. Each had the same kind of ovarian cyst. They needed surgery.

Each chose a different surgeon. The insurance company paid each doctor the same.

---

[7] Lisa and Kate are composites of women known to the authors who both went through these procedures as described.

The surgeons explained the procedure they would be using. Both had assumed they might lose an ovary as a result of the surgery, but Kate's doctor, Dr. Newway, said he thought he could save her ovary.

Dr. Oldway, Lisa's doctor, employed by an urban hospital, used a common, traditional procedure. He removed the cyst, but also removed the ovary. Her cyst, he told her later, was the size of a tennis ball. Lisa felt glad to be free of the cyst, but sad that her chances of becoming pregnant had been reduced by half.

Dr. Newway, Kate's doctor, owned an OB-GYN practice. He used a new procedure. Kate had a grapefruit-sized cyst. The new procedure left the ovary intact. Kate was glad to be free of the cyst, and very thankful to have retained a greater chance to become pregnant.

When asked why he could save Kate's ovary while Lisa's doctor could not save hers, even though Kate's cyst was twice as large as Lisa's, Dr. Newway said, "Lisa's doctor did it the old way. I do it the new way."

Which of these surgeons provided the better value? Kate and Lisa told their friends about the results of their surgery. Jenny heard them, and when she needed surgery, went to Dr. Newway.

Dr. Newway continued to be booked ahead, and

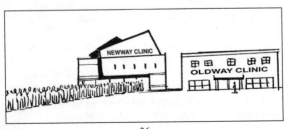

eventually increased his surgical fee. Women were willing to pay more to get the quality of results he offered.

Meanwhile, Dr. Oldway nearly went out of business. As a result, he realized he had to change. He learned the new procedure, and soon after, began advertising it at 75 percent of what Dr. Newway now charged.

Dr. Newway saw his patient load begin to drop, and so, had to drop his fee to meet Dr. Oldway's fee. The cycle of increased quality and reduced price had been completed.

The point of the story is that when doctors compete for the same patients, the quality of care increases while the price decreases. For competition to work, patients need to evaluate price and quality, to decide what the best value is for them.

This is called consumer-driven health care. No government mandate can force this kind of change onto the health care system.

THIS IS HOW PRIVATE MARKETS WORK WITHOUT GOVERNMENT INTERFERENCE

We saw Dr. Newway and Dr. Oldway competing to provide surgical services to the same group of women. The women had free choice to go to either doctor. Each doctor freely chose how to perform the procedure, and the doctors were free to charge what they knew the women would pay. The women had the freedom to pay the price they felt was the best value. This is how consumerism works.

Competition had created options. Patients demanded information about price and value, and wanted freedom to choose. The surgeons filled a need at a price the patients were willing to pay. In all this, the patient drove the market.

These are not new ideas. Rather, these are the ideas that drove health care a generation ago, when people could afford it; when hospitals could not take advantage of vulnerable people with their gotcha prices.

Remember, this consumerized health care cycle starts with one simple question, "How much does this cost?"

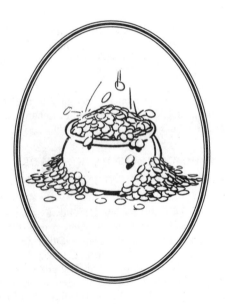

CHAPTER 8

IT'S YOUR POT OF GOLD

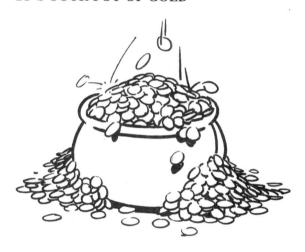

A generation ago it was normal for people to ask, "How much does this cost?" Why? Because they paid nearly half the cost of care out of their own pocket. There was no gotcha price, just the consumerized price.

That prior generation directed their own health care because they had the money to do so and costs were more affordable. Their health insurance premiums were low, because they were not paying for expensive prepaid health insurance. The insurance they bought was only to protect them from unexpected major medical expenses that could

> *"He who has the gold makes the rules."*
>
> *Economic Golden rule*

otherwise leave them in bankruptcy. Since they paid less for health insurance premiums, they had the money to direct their own health care. This is called the economic Golden Rule: He who has the gold makes the rules.

Picture yourself as the passenger in the back seat of a taxi. You tell the driver you want to get to Point X, and to take the toll road that heads downtown. But the driver takes a route down a bumpy, congested city street to save on paying tolls. The driver does this because his dispatcher told him which route to take. The dispatcher read from the driving guidelines that he received from taxi company managers.

The driver has covered up the meter so you have no idea how much the trip actually costs. Since you are paying a flat prepaid taxi fee, you don't really care: Your cost is the same.

Now picture yourself driving your own car. You are in control. You may choose to take any route to Point X. The route you choose takes you on a smooth road, it is quicker, and well worth the $2.00 toll. *You* have the gold and *you* make the rules.

Getting the health insurance gold back into your hands, as it was a generation ago, is done with consumer-driven health insurance. You keep more of your gold because you pay less expensive premiums.

Consumer-driven health insurance changes your buying behavior so that you begin asking the golden question: "How much does this cost?" Sound familiar? You demand

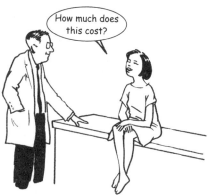

to pay the consumerized price and are no longer willing to pay the gotcha price.

The more often you demand to pay the consumerized price, the greater your pot of gold grows. What greater incentive is there than this: for you to demand a better price and greater value?

INSURANCE, NOT PREPAID HEALTH CARE

Consumer-driven health insurance works more like auto insurance.

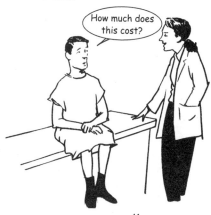

- Auto insurance protects your assets (pot of gold) from expensive, unexpected accidents and pays to repair your damaged auto body. Consumer-driven health insurance protects your assets from expensive, unexpected illness or injury, but provides money to help pay the cost of healing your body.

- You hope never to file an auto insurance claim due to a car accident. With consumer-driven health insurance, you hope never to have to file a claim due to illness or injury.

As a result of buying consumer-driven health insurance, you can often save 40 percent or more on insurance premiums compared to prepaid and traditional health insurance. What should you do with the savings? Where can you store your pot of gold, and how do you maximize its growth?

How to Increase Your Pot of Gold & Still Be Insured

You can choose to reduce your health insurance cost by 40 percent or more. Instead of sending $10,000 a year to the insurance company for prepaid health care, you can send them $6,000 for a consumer-driven health insurance policy, and save the $4,000 difference.

The $6,000 insurance policy provides peace of mind by protecting your financial assets from unforeseen major medical claims. It also gives you the security that you will be able to receive the health care you need, but at a more affordable price.

The $4,000 you no longer send to the insurance company is yours to keep. This savings is what will motivate you to replace gotcha behavior with consumerized behavior. You become extremely, enthusiastically motivated to ask, "How much does this cost?" because it's your money you are spending, not someone else's.

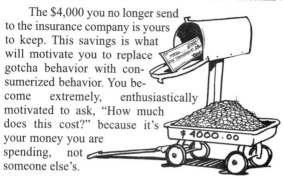

Congress and most state legislators endorse consumer-driven health insurance. They recognize it as affordable and it reduces the cost of health care. It also encourages uninsured people to purchase insurance – 33 percent of people who have recently bought this type of insurance were previously uninsured. This saves government and taxpayers billions of dollars otherwise spent to care for uninsured people.

Since 2003 the United States government, and most state governments, have been encouraging you to save money for future health expenses. You do this by depositing money into a Health Savings Account (HSA) – your pot of gold.

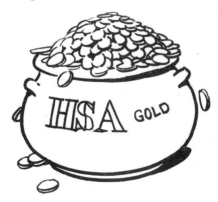

Your HSA is where you deposit the premium savings you gain from purchasing less costly insurance. The money you put into the HSA is 100 percent tax deductible, subject to annual limits. In 2009 the maximum deposit will be $3,000 for you, or $5,950 total for your family – these deposits are tax deductible. (People 55 or older can add another $1,000 a year, in what is called a catch up deposit.)[9]

If after depositing your premium savings, you have not yet reached the maximum allowable amount ($3,000 for an individual, or $5,950 for a family), you can continue to make deposits until you reach the maximum. These funds are all tax deductible.

The HSA tax deduction is easy to understand. When your employer or you (or both) deposit money into your HSA, neither you nor your employer pays taxes on that money. You will never pay taxes on that money, even if it doubles or triples in value, as long as the money taken from it is spent on eligible health related expenses such as medical, dental, vision, hearing, and other health costs.

Your professional health insurance agent can help you with the details about the HSA.

The idea behind the HSA is simple. As you spend your own money on health care (from your HSA) you will be much more careful about the price of what you purchase, and how often you spend your money. That is because the money saved on health expenses becomes part of your retirement pot of gold.

If you face a financial need for non-health related expenses, you may withdraw money from your Health Savings Account. If you do, you will have to pay taxes on it, plus a penalty. If you lose your job and the mortgage payment is due, it can bring you peace of mind.

---

[9] http://www.hsabank.com

HSA Pot of Gold is Yours to Keep

Your HSA is yours. It always will be. Use it to pay health care expenses. If you do not spend it, the money grows tax free to become part of your estate. At retirement, it could be a large pot of gold.

The HSA is your pot of gold.

HSAS LINKED TO
CONSUMER-DRIVEN HEALTH INSURANCE

HSAs are only allowed with consumer-driven health insurance policies. These have deductibles that are greater than HMO plans or prepaid insurance plans. These are usually called "high deductible health plans."

The government will not allow you to have an HSA with a prepaid insurance plan, only with consumer-driven, high deductible health plans.

By combining a Health Savings Account with a consumer-driven health plan, the government believes that you will spend your own health dollars more carefully. You will insist on paying the consumerized price, not the gotcha price. As a result, national health care spending will stabilize, or go down.

As you spend your own money on what you believe is important, competition among health providers will increase. Quality and value will improve. Everyone benefits and that is good.

Controlling health care spending happens as a result of consumer-driven health insurance, smart tax policy, personal choice and responsibility, and maximum competition. These are the keys to cure what ails health care.

And it all starts with "How much does this cost?"

SECTION III

HOW TO BUY HEALTH CARE
AND SAVE MONEY

CHAPTER 9

PROTECTING YOUR POT OF GOLD

Once you decide to purchase consumer-driven health insurance and set up your Health Savings Account, you are now ready to change your behavior to stretch each health care dollar, spending the least amount of money for the greatest amount of health care. You will be determined to no longer pay the gotcha price, but instead, to pay the consumerized price.

Let's start with prescription drugs.

HOW TO REPLACE THE $100 GOTCHA
PILL WITH THE $2 CONSUMERIZED PILL

What is a $100 Gotcha Pill? This is the prescription that costs $100, but it is bought without much thought, since you only pay a small co-pay. In the past, you focused on what the pill will do, not its cost. Now, since you have to pay for it out of your pot of your HSA, you are concerned about the price.

What is a $2 Consumerized Pill? This prescription is the same medicine, but costs $2 a month. You buy it with more thought than the Gotcha Pill. You are focused on what the pill will do, but you are also aware of what you pay for it.

"Is one pill safer than the other?" No, both are approved by the Food and Drug Administration. Their side effects mirror each other. Why? Both pills have the same ingredients.

So what is the difference between the $100 pill and $2 pill? *You*. You choose which one to buy. One is called the Gotcha Pill, and the other, the Consumerized Pill.

Okay, there is one other difference. The Gotcha Pill is a name brand pill sold by the company that created it. The original company spent hundreds of millions of dollars on research to discover the ingredients, run clinical tests, and manufacture the pill.

The Consumerized Pill is a generic version of the name brand pill, created by a competitor of the original drug company. It has the same ingredients as the name brand pill.

The generic competitor has to wait 20 years for the Gotcha Pill to lose its patent protection. But once the patent protection expires, competitors enter the market. The result of this competition is a dramatic price reduction that could save you a lot of money.

THE CONSUMERIZED PILL

Save 98% using generics. Save 95% by shopping competitors. Save 50% more with a pill splitter.

Step 1: Cutting the cost of prescription drugs starts when you first talk with your doctor. When the doctor writes your prescription he or she may write "DAW" on it. DAW means "Dispense as Written." This tells the pharmacist not to substitute a generic for a name brand drug. If the doctor does not write DAW on the prescription, the pharmacy will automatically substitute a generic, if one is available.

Step 2: If your prescription says DAW, you have the right to ask, "Are there generic alternatives?" If there are generic alternatives, you ask the doctor to explain why the name brand drug is a better option. If you are not satisfied with the answer, you can ask the doctor to rewrite the prescription without DAW written on it.

Step 3: If there is a generic: Check the internet for local pharmacies that offer discounted prices. Many discount chain stores sell a month's supply of generics for $4.00, or $10.00 for a three month supply.

Look up the phone numbers of the pharmacies in your area, and then call them. Ask "How much does this cost?"

Be ready for this question: "Who is your insurance company?" This allows the pharmacist to refuse to tell you the price. That is because the selling price depends on the contract the pharmacy has with your insurance company. The pharmacist needs the doctor's prescription in hand to process it through your insurance plan before telling you the price. To avoid this, let the pharmacist know that you want the cash price. (If you have prescription coverage, the price will be 7-15 percent less than the cash price.)

Notice the price difference in Table 1 on the next page. Chain Store 1 asked, "Who is your insurance company?" while Chain Store 2 published their cash price on the internet. We would never have known the wide price difference without finding out the price at more than one pharmacy.

You should always beware when the price is difficult to get: The Gotcha Price may be hiding behind it.

Table I
Price Comparison for Zocor and Simvastatin at Two Chain Store Pharmacies

DRUG	DOSAGE	CHAIN STORE 1[10]	CHAIN STORE 2[11]
Zocor simvastatin	20 MG	$1,786 a year	$1,757 a year
Generic simvastatin	20 MG	$729 a year	$38 a year
Zocor simvastatin	40 MG	$1,802 a year	$1,703 a year
Generic simvastatin	40 MG	$729 a year	$50 a year

[10] The actual prices retrieved by phone from a retail national chain store, Friday, August 8, 2008
[11] The actual prices selected from the website of a national discount store, Friday, August 8, 2008.

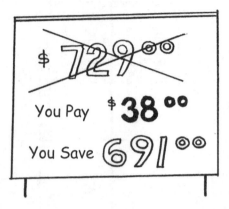

A REAL EXAMPLE OF SAVING A LOT OF GOLD

Let's use 20 mg of generic simvastatin, a common dosage (one per day) for our example. In Table 1 you see that Chain Store 1 charges $729 for a year's supply, while Chain Store 2 charges just $38. Buy it at Chain Store 2 and you save $691 from your pot of gold by just asking, "How much does this cost?" and persisting in getting the answer.

Many pills can be split in two. If you buy the 40 mg simvastatin at Chain Store 2 and split the pills, you can save another $13. In this way, a year's supply of simvastatin will cost you just $25, and that is 98.6 percent less than the cost of Zocor, the 20 mg Gotcha Pill, at Chain Store 1.

NAME BRAND ONLY: THERE STILL COULD BE A WAY TO PROTECT YOUR POT OF GOLD

If there is no generic alternative for a Gotcha Pill, pill splitting becomes more important. Ask your doctor to prescribe a dosage that is twice what you are to take; then split the pills in half. For example, by purchasing 40 mg Zocor at Chain Store 2, the cost drops from $1,757 (20

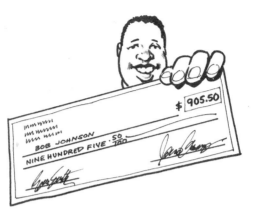

mg) to $851.50 after you split 40 mg tablets in two (half of $1,703). This saves you $905.50, more than 50 percent. Pill splitting takes effort, but it pays high wages. Splitting a 90-day supply of pills takes 15 minutes. Do it four times a year, and you earn $905.50 an hour. This kind of savings can easily become habit-forming, but it is a good habit, not a costly bad habit.

IF YOU CANNOT AFFORD
TO PAY FOR YOUR MEDICINE

The pharmaceutical industry is aware that their medicines are expensive, and that some people cannot afford them. They have created a website to help people find affordable medicines. If you or someone you know needs financial help to buy medicines, go to:

https://www.pparx.org/Intro.php

CHAPTER 10

HOW TO REPLACE THE $1,000 GOTCHA VISIT WITH THE $60-$200 CONSUMERIZED VISIT

What is a $1,000 Gotcha Visit? This is when you go to an emergency room (ER) without much thought. You do this out of habit, and are focused on urgency, not the cost. You expect your insurance to pay for most of it.

What is a $60-$200 Consumerized Visit? This office visit costs $60-$200, but is bought with more thought than the Gotcha Visit. You are focused on what the visit will do, but you are also aware of what it costs, because you may pay for it from your HSA pot of gold.

So what is the difference between the $1,000 Gotcha Visit and the $60-$200 Consumerized Visit? *You*. You make the choice of which to buy.

Okay. There are other differences.

•   Gotcha Clinics (ERs) are designed to deal with extreme, life-threatening situations. These are the emergencies that might happen once or twice in a lifetime. They sometimes require an ambulance ride. Inside the ambulance you give no thought to the cost: And that makes sense.

•   When you go to the ER, you usually get many more tests. Soon that $1,000 ER visit explodes in cost to thousands of dollars more: an

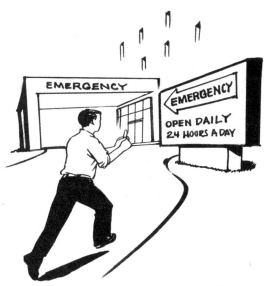

MRI, a stress test, blood work, X-rays, maybe a questionable stay overnight in the hospital.

When you seriously feel that your life is threatened you should go to the ER. For non-life-threatening problems there are better choices. These are the minor emergencies that can be treated at an Urgent Care Center. Not only will you save money and get excellent service, you will also reduce the misery of sitting and waiting in a hospital ER.

WHY WE BUY THE $1,000 GOTCHA VISIT

Emergency rooms are misused because someone else pays most of the cost. In fact, many insurance policies actually make it attractive to use the ER by insulating you from the true cost. You may pay $50, $75, or a $100 co-pay; the insurance company pays $900 or more. This cost is passed on to you with higher insurance premiums.

For the Gotcha Price, you would think that the ER would provide short wait times. For most people, however, an ER visit takes four to eight hours. Why? Federal law requires hospitals to treat everyone that comes to the ER, even the uninsured. And many insured people go to the ER with nothing but a runny nose, the flu, or a fever. This slows down service for everyone.

Now that you are interested in protecting your pot of gold, you ask, "Why am I going to the ER, spending all this money, and having to wait so long? There's got to be a better way." There is.

Urgent Care Centers:
the $60-$200 Consumerized Visit for
non-life threatening emergencies

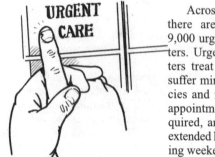

Across the country there are more than 9,000 urgent care centers. Urgent care centers treat people who suffer minor emergencies and illnesses. No appointment is required, and they offer extended hours, including weekends.

Urgent care centers offer quicker service at a reduced cost. Wait times at urgent care centers are far shorter than at the ER. They are staffed by doctors, provide safe and effective care, and are more convenient. If your condition is a serious emergency, urgent care centers are prepared to quickly move you to a hospital ER.

The greatest motivator to change buying behavior

(between urgent care and the ER) is what you have to pay. If you pay out of your pot of gold, you will prefer the consumerized clinic – urgent care. Yet, you will still get the services you need.

You can learn more at http://www.urgentcare.org/. You can find the closest urgent care center at http://www.DexKnows.com or www.usdirectory.com. Your health insurance company will be glad to help you find the closest urgent care center to your home or business. Post this information in your home and at work, where you can find it when you need it.

How to save 75 percent by using a Consumerized Office Visit

Competition for your health care dollar has created yet another affordable alternative. Retail walk-in health clinics all across the country provide basic health services at very low cost. These retail clinics are conveniently located in grocery stores, shopping centers, pharmacies, and elsewhere.

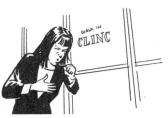

Retail walk-in clinics are staffed by registered nurses, nurse practitioners, or physician assistants. Some clinics have doctors on staff. These professionals are highly educated and skilled to treat many common ailments and skin conditions. They offer wellness and preventive care, vaccines, and laboratory tests. These are the services that you might otherwise receive at a doctor's office.

Walk-in clinics are usually priced 25-50 percent less than what a doctor charges. When compared to an ER visit for the flu, you could save 75 percent.

For more information and to locate a walk in clinic, go to http://www.convenientcareassociation.org/ or call your insurance company.

TOOLS TO INCREASE
QUALITY AND REDUCE PRICE

We live in the information age, and there is no shortage of health care information easily available to you at no cost. You can use this information to manage your own

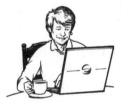

health care. This will allow you to control your cost and to partner with the doctor. The result will be better outcomes and more value for your health care dollars.

The internet includes hundreds of websites that:

- Explain a medical condition, to help you understand and manage it.

- Help you to attempt to diagnose your own health condition.

- Help you find the best quality doctors.

- Show which hospitals excel in the type of care you need.

- Show the price of health services before you buy them.

- Allow you to order medical products, devices, and medicines at a discount.

- Allow you to monitor your Health Savings Account and health insurance.

- Allow you to securely store your health records online.

Health insurance companies feature user-friendly websites. State and federal government websites overflow with information. Your health insurance agent will be more than willing to guide you through this maze of information.

FOR LOW-INCOME, UNINSURED PEOPLE

For low-income people who may not be able to afford urgent care or even a retail walk-in clinic, there is a great alternative. It is far better than an emergency room.

> … community health centers provide vital primary care to more than 17 million Americans with limited financial resources…health centers focus on meeting the basic health care needs of their individual communities. Health centers maintain an open-door policy, providing treatment regardless of an individual's income or insurance coverage.

> Health centers serve the homeless, residents of public housing, migrant farm workers and others with emergent and chronic health care needs, but limited resources to secure treatment through traditional channels.[12]

There are more than 1,150 Community Health Centers (CHCs) across the United States. These are located in or near every community. You can find the CHC nearest to you by going online and entering your zip code at:

http://findahealthcenter.hrsa.gov/

The fact is that in the United States, everyone, regardless of their ability to pay, can get preventive and corrective health care. While a CHC may not provide comprehensive care such as at the Mayo Clinic, they do offer a complete mix of high quality services.

---

[12] http://www.nachc.com/about-our-health-centers.cfm

CHAPTER 11

CONSUMERIZING
HOSPITAL GOTCHA PRICES

In any given year, 92 percent of Americans spend $0-$1,000 on health care.[13] These dollars are for routine, minor health issues, and screenings; the kind that require seeing a family doctor or nurse practitioner. We showed you how changing your behavior preserved your pot of gold when buying these services.

About eight percent of Americans spend a good deal of money on health care each year.[13] These are people with chronic or sudden illness, or who are injured, and those in their last months of life. These people consume a large volume of health services, and oftentimes in a hospital. Hospital care is by far the most expensive kind of care – and as we've shown, the most outrageously priced.

HOSPITALS HAVE CHANGED

The Centers for Medicare and Medicaid Services have shown us that hospitals grossly overcharge. They charge 308 percent more for services than what they know Medicare will pay them. Hospitals tell us they cannot make money on what Medicare pays them, but is this true? "The Medicare payment is designed by law to pay a little more than the cost incurred by an efficiently run hospital."[14]

---

[13] Hopper, R., & Hopper, D. (2007). Healthcare Happily Ever After. Overland Park, KS: A.D. Banker & Company, LLC.
[14] Rooney, P., & Perrin, D. (2008). America's health care crisis solved. Hoboken, New Jersey: John Wiley & Sons, Inc.

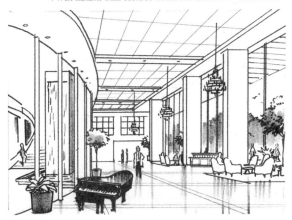

When profit margins are tight, like with Medicare payments, hospitals are forced to be efficient. But when hospitals charge the gotcha price to everyone not on Medicare or Medicaid, they do not have to be efficient; they waste health care dollars, and build extravagant facilities.

In most locations, hospitals negotiate with insurance companies to be paid at a rate of 25-50 percent greater than the Medicare rate. And those hospitals charge uninsured people 308 percent or more than the Medicare rate.

Earlier, we told you that one of this book's authors had a nuclear stress test during August 2008, and the hospital billed his insurance company $6,106 for the test. If the author had been uninsured, the hospital would have chased him down for the full amount. His insurance company, however, allowed the hospital to charge only $1,188, $4,918 less than the gotcha price.

The author is glad that the insurance company negotiated a realistic price for all of their policyholders to protect them from the gotcha price. The hospital would never have accepted $1,188 if it wasn't enough to generate a profit. Why, then, can't the hospital accept that amount from everyone who has a nuclear stress test?

Why try to charge $6,106 for a service only worth $1,188? No other product or service in the United States is priced this way. You would never allow a business that charged this way to stay in business. You demand honest, transparent pricing, except for health care. You, and all of us, can change this. Let's see how.

IF YOU GET A GOTCHA BILL

What would you do if you received a $6,106 gotcha bill for a test that should cost no more than $1,188? What would you do if the hospital hired attorneys to track you down and demanded that you pay the gotcha price? Can you do anything to protect your pot of gold from this price gouging?

Yes. There are strategies you can use to negotiate a fair price.

One strategy is to use the media. Hospitals are sensitive about how communities perceive them. They want to be seen as caring, compassionate institutions.

Hospitals do not want the community to know they charge the gotcha price, making a windfall profit on local citizens. They especially worry about being accused of gouging the uninsured. The media loves sensational stories about large institutions that take advantage of their viewers. Let them know that the hospital is trying to take advantage of you, and the reporters will beat a path to your door.

STRATEGY TO NEGOTIATE

The good news is, we can stop paying the gotcha price to hospitals. Here is how:

Step 1: When at all possible, ask "How much does

this cost?" before using a hospital's services. Also ask for the price paid by people without insurance.

<u>Step 2</u>: Ask how much Medicare allows the hospital to charge for the same service.

<u>Step 3</u>: Ask your insurance company how much they allow the hospital to charge, based on your insurance plan.

The authors at random checked out Northwest Community Hospital, in Arlington Heights, Illinois.[14] We looked at this hospitals charges for "Ancillary Services," specifically for "Radiology-Diagnostic." There we found that Northwest Community Hospital charges 638 percent more than its cost while Johns Hopkins, the prestigious Maryland hospital, charges only 103 percent more than its cost. If Northwest Community Hospital charged the author $6,106 for a nuclear stress test, then the real price should have been $957 (based on Johns Hopkins' pricing structure).

If your hospital billed you $6,106 for a service that should cost no more than $957, would you be upset? Would you be willing to demand a reduced price – the consumerized price?

<u>Step 4</u>: Negotiate a price based on no more than 125 percent above Medicare allowance.

Here are some easy steps to take, if you believe your hospital is price-gouging:

1.   Call your insurance agent and ask for help.

---

[14] The cost data for this example was taken from http://www.hospitalvictims.org/Pages/Illinois_hospital_prices/Arlington_Heights/Northwest_Community_Hospital.htm. The website is no longer available there, but can be viewed at http://www.freemarkethealthcare.com/whycost.htm. The negotiating procedures likewise came from hospitalvictims.org, and are available at the freemarkethealthcare.com website as above.

2. Write a letter to the editor of your newspaper and date it two weeks later. Ask the hospital to favorably resolve the bill with you, and let them know, if they do not, you will send the letter.

3. At the same time you send the letter, call a local radio or TV news department.

4. Send copies of your letter to elected officials that represent you.

5. Email your friends.

6. Tell your neighbors.

Remember, you are not at fault here. While you *do* owe the hospital for their services, you should not allow them to take advantage of you with the gotcha price.

IF THEIR COLLECTION
ATTORNEYS PURSUE YOU

If you are being pursued by a collection firm because of outrageous hospital charges, go to http://www.freemarkethealthcare.com/hospitals.htm and click onto "Defend Yourself."[14] It will provide step-by-step, easily understood information on what to do. You have rights, but you need to know how to exercise them.

The website will show you how to write a letter to the hospital and their law firm to stop them from harassing you.

Testimony from leading hospital authorities claim that a hospital should be willing to settle for 25 percent above what Medicare pays. In other words, if Medicare pays a hospital $1,000 for a service, you should pay no more than $1,250.

In a lawsuit against BayCare Health System, Tampa,

Florida, the court ordered the hospital to accept 20 percent above Medicare as its full payment for services.[15] Therefore, if you must settle an outrageous hospital bill, you should pay no more than 20-25 percent above what Medicare allows for the same service.

If you have private health insurance, you should still be vitally concerned about how much your insurance company pays the hospital. Ultimately, those charges will end up increasing your insurance premium.

WHERE ARE THE POLITICIANS?

Why have politicians tolerated hospital price gouging for their constituents? Maybe it has to do with the political power hospitals enjoy, or maybe politicians haven't heard from enough people like you; but they should.

You should have the right to know the price of anything you buy; especially health care. Some leading states have laws that require price "transparency." Transparency means that a health care provider must tell you the price it will charge you, if you ask before services are rendered. This estimate includes how much your insurance company will allow them to charge, based on your health plan. This may or may not be true in your state, but it should be.

The most aggressive price transparency law protecting consumers from provider price gouging requires a "Good Faith Estimate." This is similar to laws that require auto service stations to tell you how much repairs will cost prior to doing the work. Health care price transparency Good Faith Estimates require the provider to tell you what they will charge for a particular service. Of course, if they find some unknown complication, they can charge you

---

[15] Rooney, P., & Perrin, D. (2008). America's health care crisis solved. Hoboken, New Jersey: John Wiley & Sons, Inc.

more. But the fact that they have to tell you the price ahead of time will have the effect, over time, of reducing the price.

Find a copy of Minnesota's transparency law at: http://www.freemarkethealthcare.com/transparency.htm. If you, and thousands of others like you, write to the politicians, they will listen. Write your Congressman and state legislator. We have provided sample letters on the website at http://www.freemarketheatlhcare.com/sampleletters.htm.

WHAT OTHER ROLE SHOULD GOVERNMENT PLAY?

Americans have shown through ongoing funding of government health care programs that we are a compassionate people. We wish to help low-income people to get the health care they need. And we know that many retired citizens need help paying for health care. This is why federal and state governments have a role in paying for health care through Medicare, Medicaid, and other programs.

Today's government health plans are shrouded in secrecy, overly complex, and require an army of government bureaucrats and third party administrators to make them work. There is a better and less costly way to provide health care for people using government programs or people who are uninsured. We write about this in another book like this one: *Why health care costs so much: The Solution-Governments' Role.* To find out about this book, send an email to alethospress@comcast.net.

CHAPTER 12

A SENSIBLE HEALTH INSURANCE POLICY

The United States has a vibrant private health insurance system in addition to government health care plans. Private insurance paid $725 billion for health care for Americans in 2007. It is one of our nation's strengths.

If Americans choose to do away with private health insurance, and move toward a government-run health system, what would happen to that $725 billion? Without it, we would face third-world health care. Or, we would ask politicians to raise taxes by at least $725 billion a year so we can get the health care we want. But they would not stop there; it is their nature to expand programs to win votes. Soon, $725 billion will become $1.5 trillion, or more. How would you feel about an annual tax increase of $2,417 for yourself, and each person in your family? Or, if the tax doubled, an annual increase of $4,824 each?

There is a better way, and it relies on old-fashioned American ingenuity, and citizens taking control of their own lives.

America needs a new type of health insurance policy. We believe it should have these features:

- Premiums would be affordable, predictable, and stable over the long term.

- You could go to any doctor you choose any where in the country.

- It would protect you from the Gotcha Price.

- You could control your own spending decisions, and be able to save money by paying the consumerized price.

- You would be financially rewarded for staying healthy, and have the coverage you need if you become ill or injured.

- You could set aside tax-free money in your own Health Savings Account.

There is a health plan design under development that can do all of this. It takes advantage of the way Medicare currently pays for health care. Surprisingly, it is based on the same principle we are already using; it is nothing new. But what is new is that it makes the cost of services transparent to you, not hidden like it is now. This is how it works:

Medicare pays for health services for people aged 65 and older based on a schedule. The Medicare payment schedule sets an amount that health care providers receive for the services they provide. For instance, the schedule might specify that Medicare will pay the provider $5,000 for an appendectomy.

This same Medicare schedule is used by insurance companies who insure people under age 65. They use the same Medicare schedule to determine the amount that they will pay to the same health care providers. The insurance company tries to get the provider to accept the same payment that Medicare pays, but this is seldom possible. In most locations, the amount the insurance company pays is greater than what Medicare will pay; 125-200 percent more. If the insurance company pays 150 percent above Medicare, it would pay $7,500 for the $5,000 Medicare appendectomy.

The new insurance policy would pay providers a set

percentage above Medicare's scheduled payment. The percentage could be 125 percent, 150 percent or perhaps, 200 percent. The lower the percent above Medicare, the lower will be your cost of premium.

You would always know the price of the health care you receive, because it is fully transparent. All providers already know how much Medicare pays them. It would be easy enough for them to disclose their price to you when you ask, "How much does this cost?"

This new insurance policy would eliminate provider networks. No longer would you be restricted to doctors in a network, because there would be no networks. You would be free to choose any doctor you wished that would accept you as a patient.

This would encourage competition among doctors. They would be freed from the restrictions of practicing in mega-networks and supersized clinics. They could make their own decisions, work on a personal level with you, and enjoy the practice of medicine once again. You could actually witness the re-emergence of small neighborhood medical clinics.

Doctors and hospitals would begin to price their services more competitively. They would find a way to live on a rate 25-50 percent above Medicare's rates, or even less when enough doctors compete for your business. They could reduce their administrative cost because they would no longer need to negotiate contracts with insurance companies, and that would reduce your cost of care.

Many more insurance companies would compete for your business, and the competition would drive down the cost of insurance. This savings, enjoyed by both the insurance company and the providers, comes from eliminating the huge expense of constantly negotiating contracts with every individual clinic and hospital.

Having a larger number of companies competing for your insurance dollars would reduce the cost.

This kind of insurance would produce price stability. That is because Medicare payments tend to remain flat and follow general inflation. When they do increase, it is only after a prolonged and careful review; it is gradual and predictable. Therefore, the premium for this type of health insurance policy would remain affordable over time.

We believe that the most cost-efficient and sensible health insurance plan would feature reimbursements paid to providers based on a percentage above Medicare reimbursements.

To make these policies even more valuable, they would be tied to Health Savings Accounts, and be consumer-directed. You would be able to save money tax-free, have the absolute security that your health care needs will be covered, and pay the consumerized price, not the gotcha price.

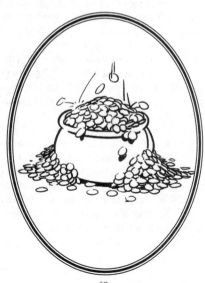

CONCLUSION

YOU ARE IN CHARGE

So why does health care cost so much?

At the beginning of this book we promised to explain why health care costs so much, and we promised to show you a solution. The solution would lead to less spending, more quality, and a better value for your hard-earned health care dollars.

Maybe you were surprised to learn this fact: *You* are the answer to the question, and *you* are the solution to the problem.

As with most issues in the United States, so it is with health care. Free people like you get to decide how they want to live, and how to spend their own money. No longer do you need to sit in the back seat, letting someone else decide how to spend your health care dollar. Remember, these are your dollars, and no one can spend your dollars more efficiently than you.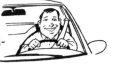

So, the solution starts with you.

Once you decide that you want to control your own health care, the health care providers, insurance companies, and politicians become your servants, not your masters. You will be surprised. Providers and insurance companies actually like it when you are actively involved in solving your own health care issues.

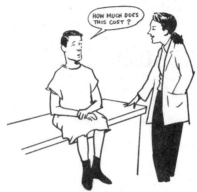

THE STARTING POINT –
HEALTHIER FINANCES

Every time a provider makes a recommendation, ask, "How much does this cost?" Then, you ask for wise counsel on how best to spend your health care dollars to get the best possible results. You want value for your money and quality services for your body.

Tell the insurance company that you want to control more of your own money. Ask your health insurance agent to enroll you in a high deductible health plan and a Health Savings Account (HSA). Ask the agent the best way to fund your HSA.

If you receive health care from an employer, ask your employer to install a high deductible health plan with a Health Savings Account.

If you do not have a health insurance agent, or your employer needs help locating one, go to:
http://www.nahu.org or http://www.ahia.net.

These are organizations of professional health insurance agents, and they will help you find an agent in your geographic area.

Do not forget the politicians. They are busy trying to find ways to solve your health care problems (or meddling with your health and freedom – it depends on your perspective). Tell them to find ways to maximize consumer-driven health care, expand the use of tax-preferred HSAs, and protect you from gotcha prices.

Let the politicians know that you want the right to examine health care charges before you use services. Tell them that, since you pay the Medicare and Medicaid taxes, you also want to be able to access how much they pay for services – transparency.

Though they seldom act like it, except at election time, politicians work for you. They are supposed to meet your needs. Let them know, and ask your neighbors to join with you.

A HEALTHIER YOU

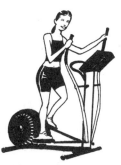

Becoming more physically fit benefits you today by making it more likely you will remain healthy tomorrow. It also means that as you age, you will be less bothered by chronic illnesses that require painful, bothersome, and expensive medical care.

If you need advice on how to get started, or to create a program that will fit your needs, call your insurance agent. Your insurance company may allow premium reductions or offer promotions in your area.

Do an Internet search on the term "wellness." The sheer number of resources will overwhelm you, but you are certain to find the help you need.

Public libraries and bookstores overflow with information about personal health and wellness.

THE UNITED STATES – LAND OF THE FREE

Reducing health care cost and improving its quality is in your hands. Health care costs so much because Americans have entrusted their health care decisions to others. You can change that for yourself, and others will follow.

Our Founders believed that you are capable of living your own life and making wise decisions, rather than entrusting your life to a government health care agency. That is why the United States is called "The land of the free and home of the brave."

Be healthier, happier, and wealthier. Ask, "How much does it cost?" That is the solution.

MORE HELP IS ON THE WAY

Changing the U.S. health system so that it answers to consumers is a big job. It requires reforming many sectors of the health care system, *and with your help, we can make that happen*. That is why we will be releasing a series of books all titled *Why health care costs so much: The Solution.* Each one will focus on a different sector, as you will see in the list below.

Government's Role.

Health Care Providers.

Employers.

Insurance Companies.

The Faith Community.

Send an email to alethospress@comcast.net for more information, or send a card or letter to:

Alethos Press LLC
PO Box 600160
St Paul, MN 55106

To Contact the Authors

Greg Dattilo and Dave Racer can be contacted by writing or emailing Alethos Press LLC:

Alethos Press LLC
P.O. Box 600160
St. Paul, MN 55106

Email: alethospress@comcast.net

The authors' biographical sketches are found at:

http://www.freemarkethealthcare.com/presskit.htm

The authors regularly speak across the country on issues addressed in this book. Use the address or email above to inquire about how you might secure them to speak for your group.

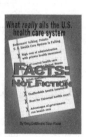
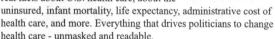

REORDERING THIS BOOK

Reordering this book can be done by clipping, or copying, and then completing **this coupon and the information on the next page**, and mailing it to the address below. Order online at the website:

http://www.alethospress.com/whycost.htm

Copy Quantity	Price Ea.	Total Bk Cst	Shipping
Bundle of 1000 copies	$1.00 ea	$1,000.00	$45.00
Bundle of 500 copies	$1.50 ea	$750.00	$39.95
Bundle of 250 copies	$1.75 ea	$437.50	$34.95
Bundle of 100 copies	$2.00 ea	$200.00	$19.95
Bundle of 50 copies	$2.25 ea	$112.50	$22.50
Bundle of 25 copies	$2.50 ea	$62.50	$9.50
Bundle of 10 copies	$3.00 ea	$30.00	$5.45
Single copy	$3.50 ea	$3.50	$2.75

Please ship _____ copies for a total of $_____

    Shipping Charges $_____

    Sub-Total $_____

    Minnesotans include sales tax at 6.5% $_____

Total Enclosed: **$**_____

Be sure to enter your contact and shipping information on the next page.

Please ship the enclosed order to:

Name: _____

Organization:_____

Address:_____

_____

City _____ St _____ Zip _____

Phone:_____

Email:_____

**Make Checks Payable To:
Alethos Press LCC**

Mail to:

**ALETHOS PRESS LLC
P.O. BOX 600160
ST. PAUL, MN 55106**

Office: 651.340.1911